my
five
senses

BY ALIKI

The world of the child is a world of discovery. He smells the odor of new-mown hay, of roses, perfume, and burning leaves. He sees blue sky, air-planes overhead, green grass, insects flitting from plant to plant. He tastes chocolate, peanuts, apples; he hears the chatter of birds, the whin-ing of a siren. His tactile sense is especially sensitive: he is able to discern delicate variations in texture. Each sound and taste, odor, sight, and touch is new and different.

Aliki captures the excitement of such discoveries in this delightful book. With simple words and sparkling pictures she develops the child's understanding of his senses, what they are and what he learns through them about the world around him.

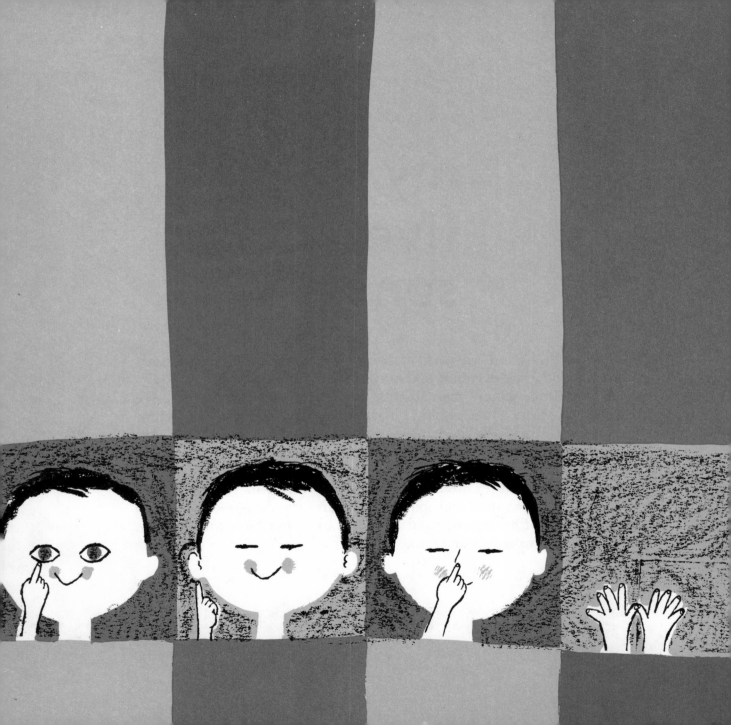

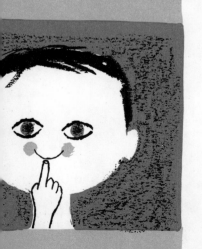

my
five
senses

by aliki

Thomas Y. Crowell Company
New York

This Crowell Crocodile is one of the quality paperback editions
selected from Crowell's highly recommended:

~ LET'S-READ-AND-FIND-OUT SCIENCE BOOKS ~

Editors: Dr. Roma Gans, Professor Emeritus of Childhood Education, Teachers College, Columbia University
Dr. Franklyn M. Branley, Astronomer Emeritus and former Chairman of the American Museum—Hayden Planetarium

L. C. Card 62-7150   ISBN 0-690-56768-5

2   3   4   5   6   7   8   9   10

CROWELL CROCODILE EDITION, 1972

my
five
senses

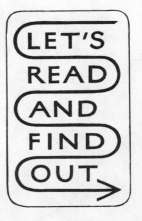

LET'S
READ
AND
FIND
OUT →

I can see! I see with my eyes.

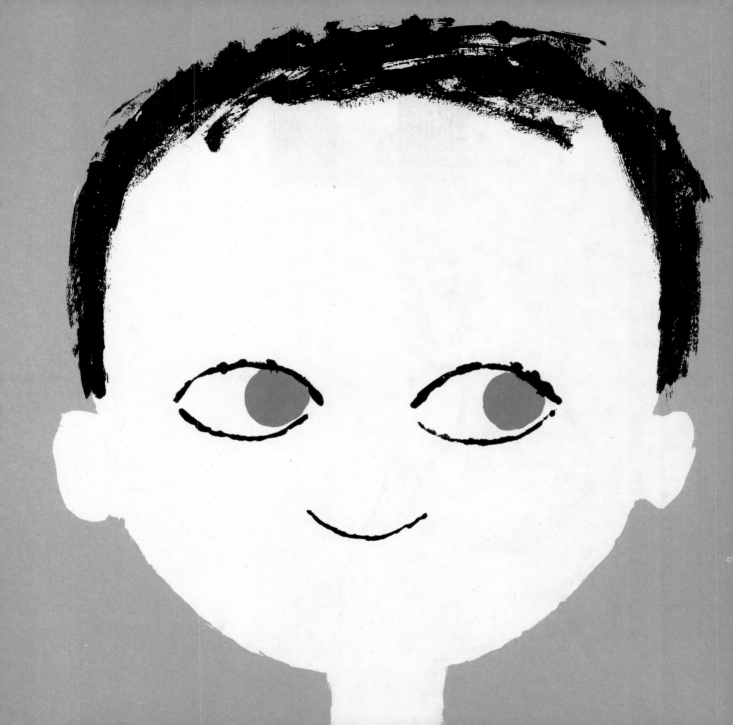

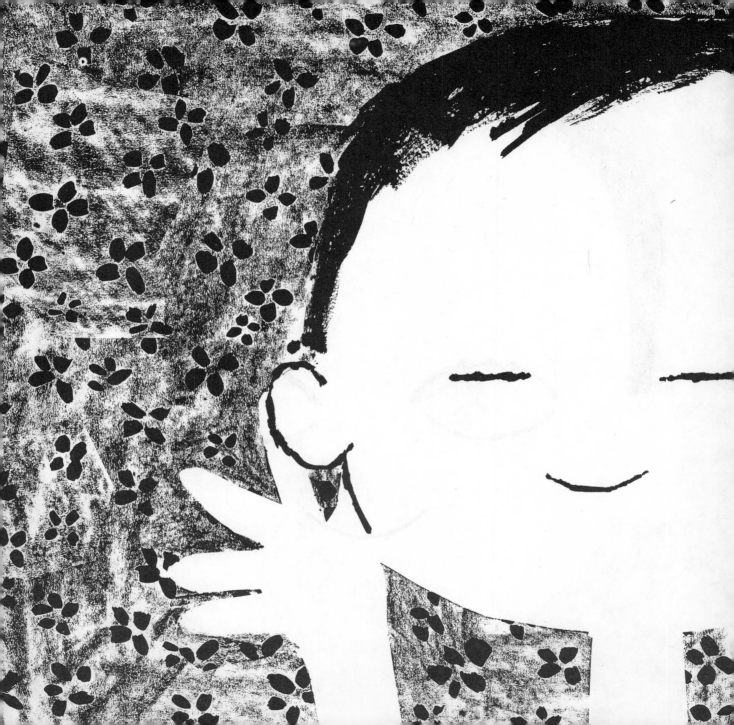

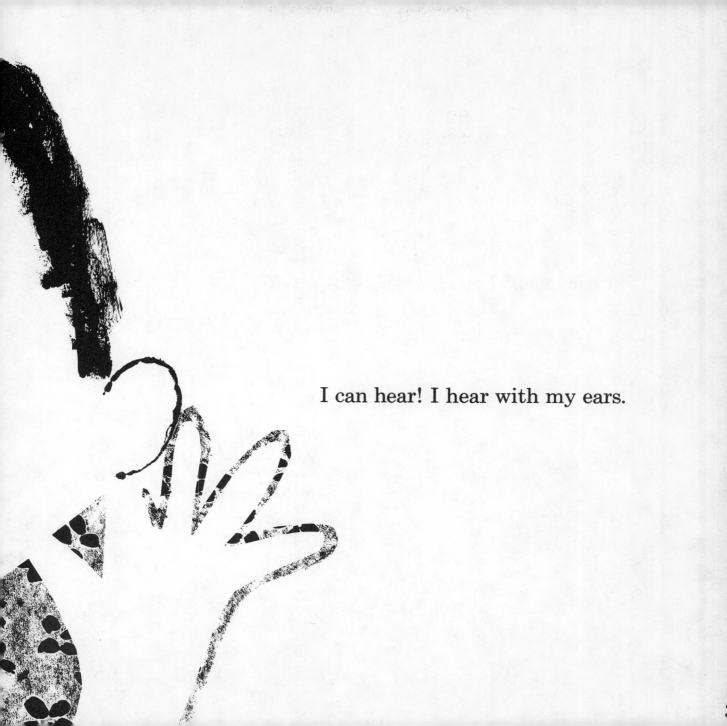

I can hear! I hear with my ears.

I can smell! I smell with my nose.

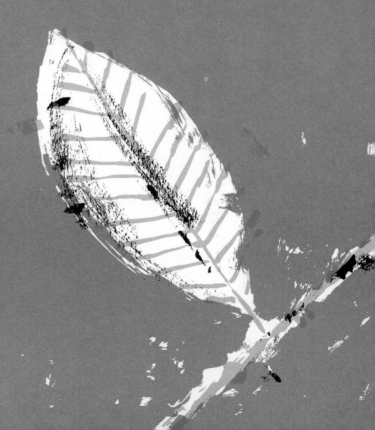

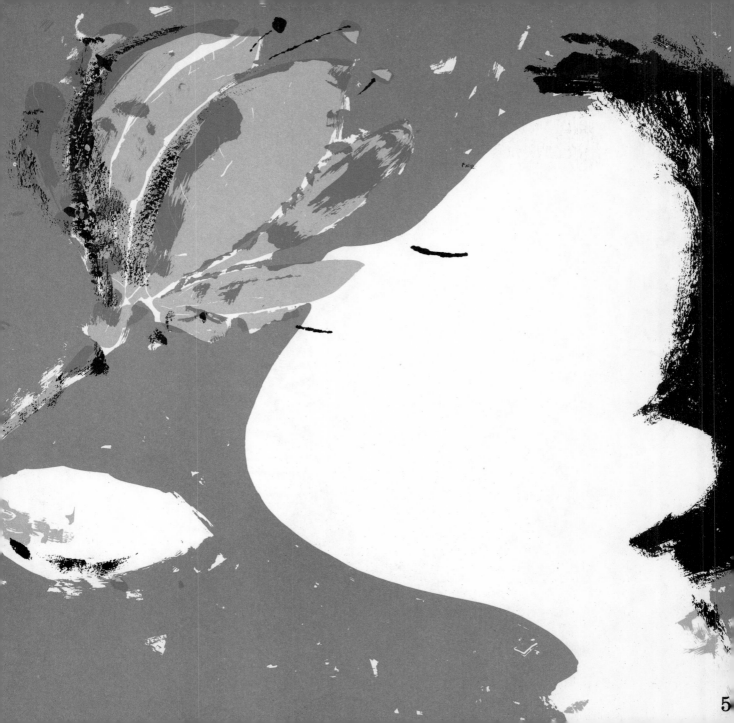

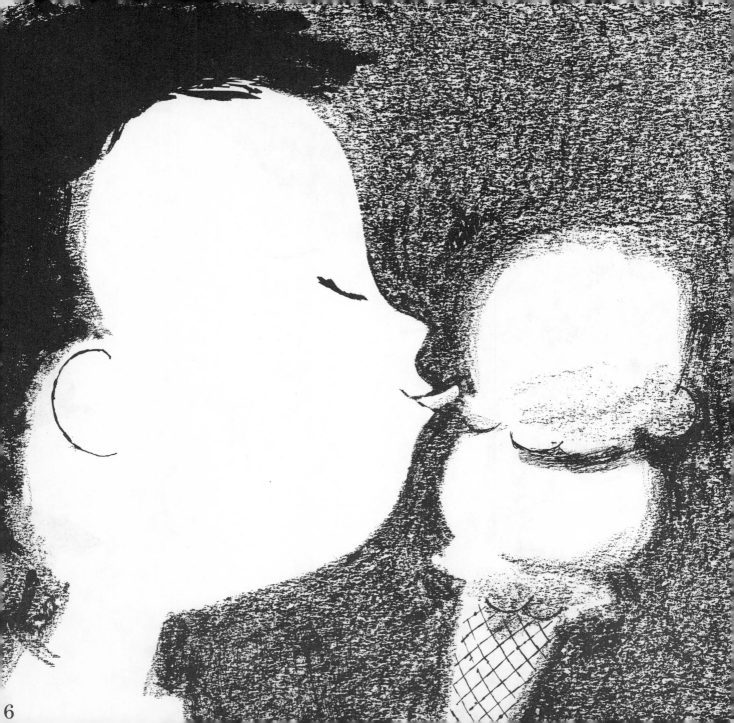

I can taste! I taste with my tongue.

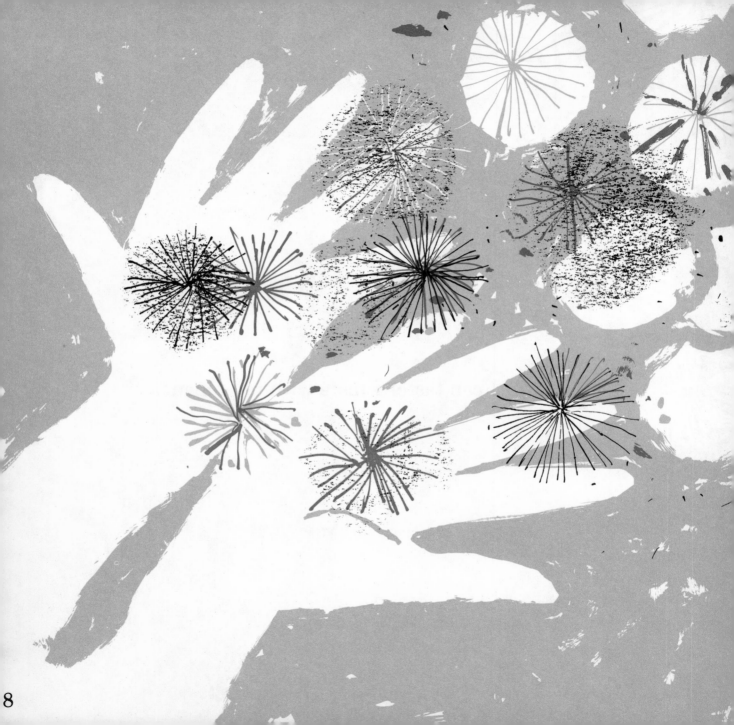

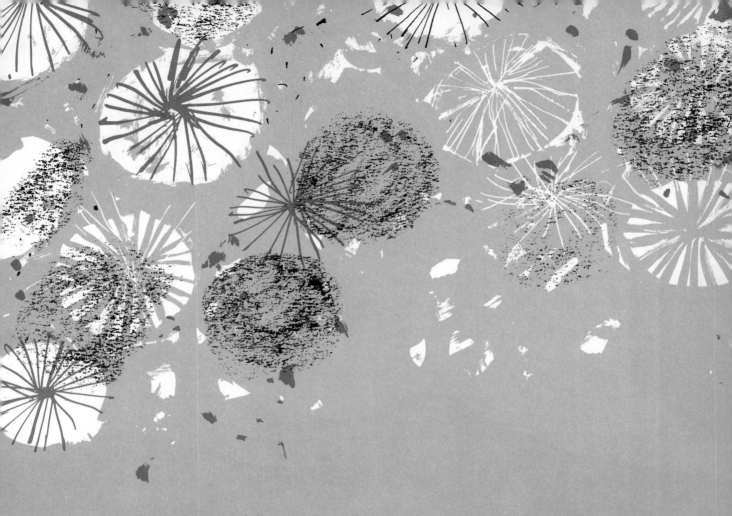

I can touch! I touch with my fingers.

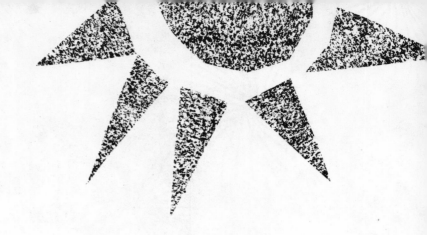

I do all this with my senses.
I have five senses.

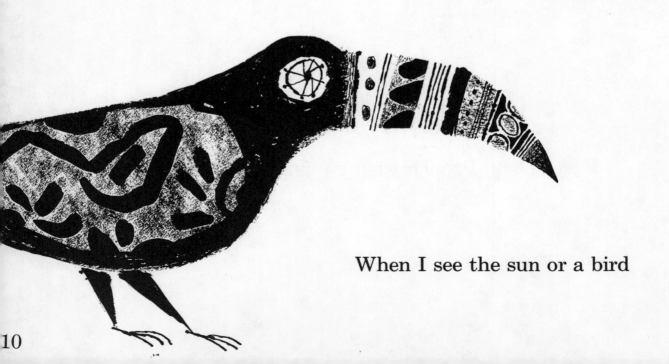

When I see the sun or a bird

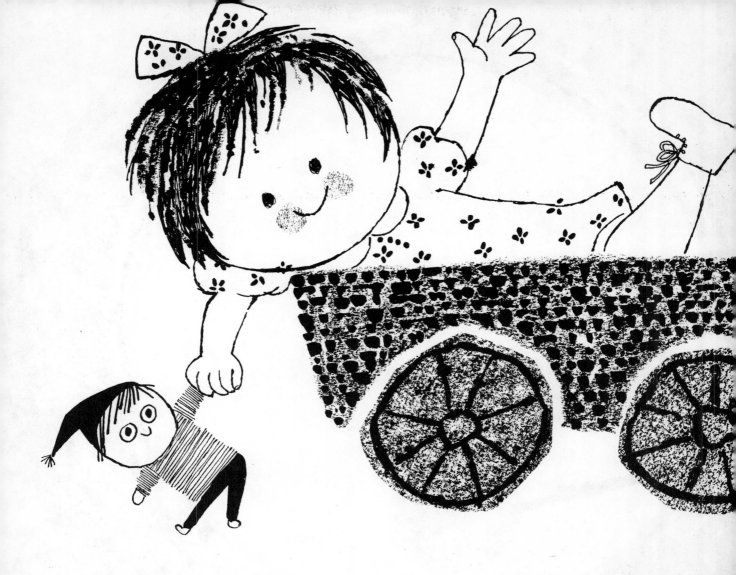

or my baby sister,
I use my sense of sight. I am seeing.

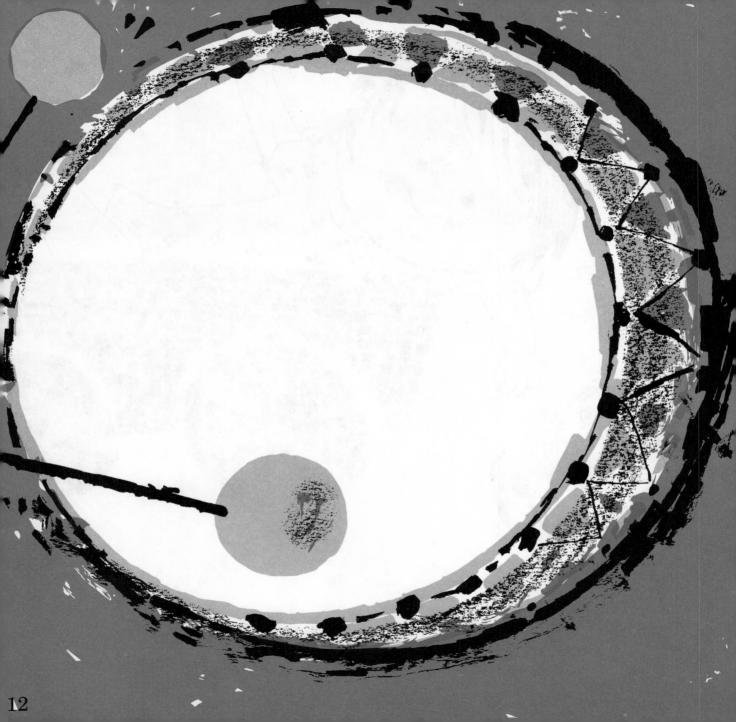

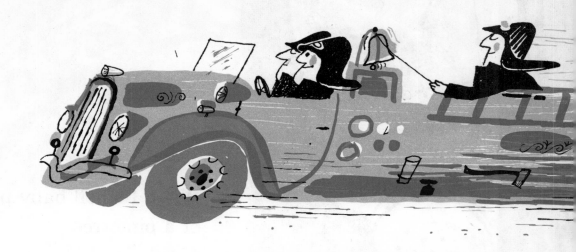

When I hear a drum or a fire engine or an egg beater,
I use my sense of sound. I am hearing.

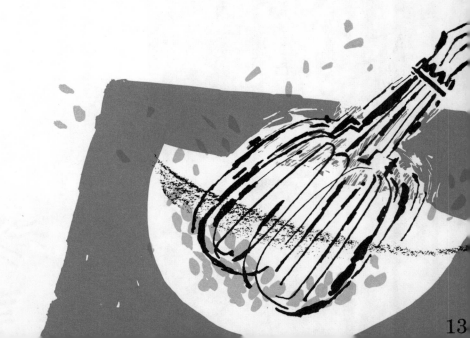

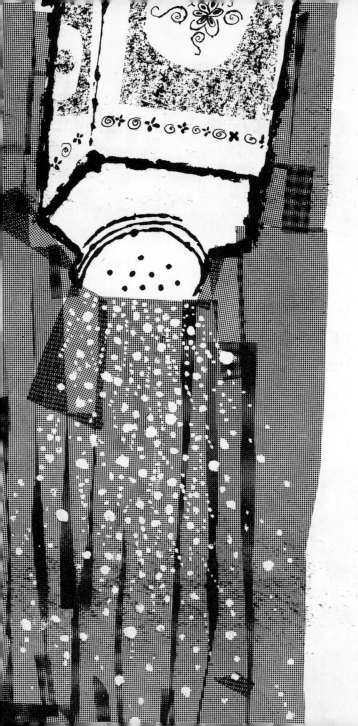

When I smell baby powder
or a pine tree

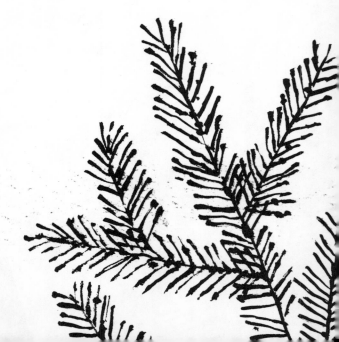

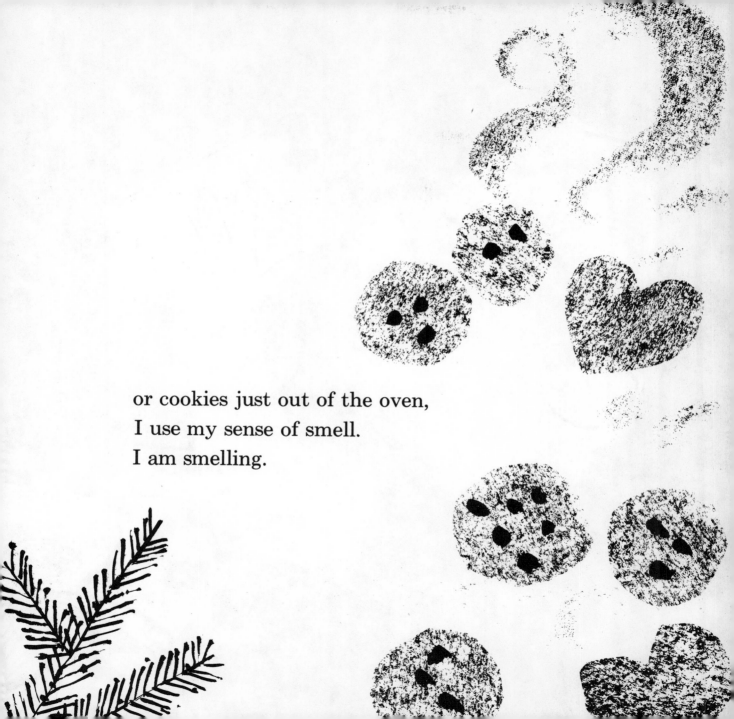

or cookies just out of the oven,
I use my sense of smell.
I am smelling.

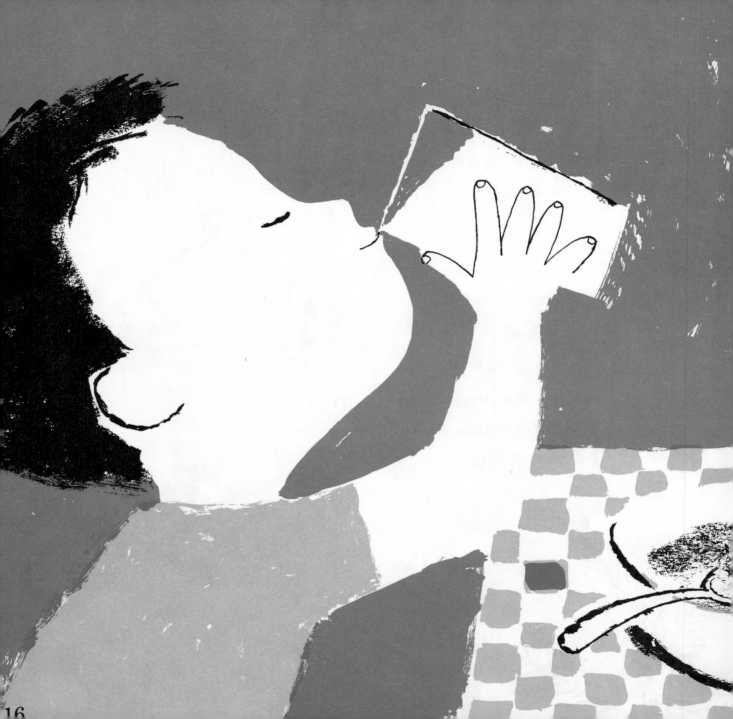

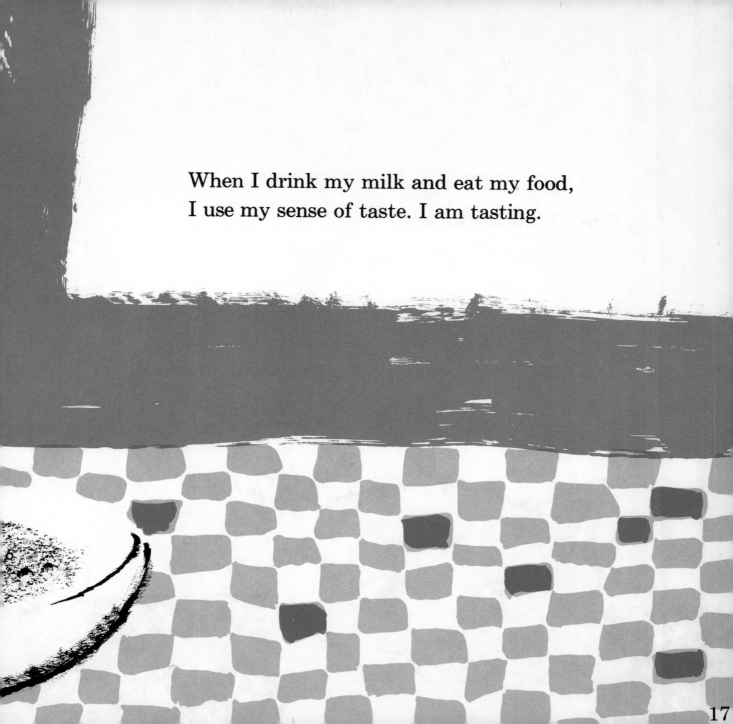

When I drink my milk and eat my food,
I use my sense of taste. I am tasting.

17

When I touch a kitten

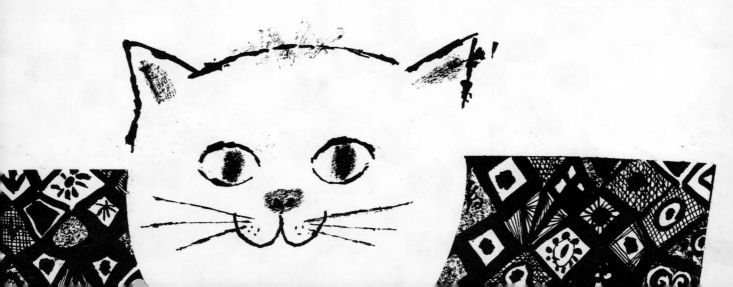

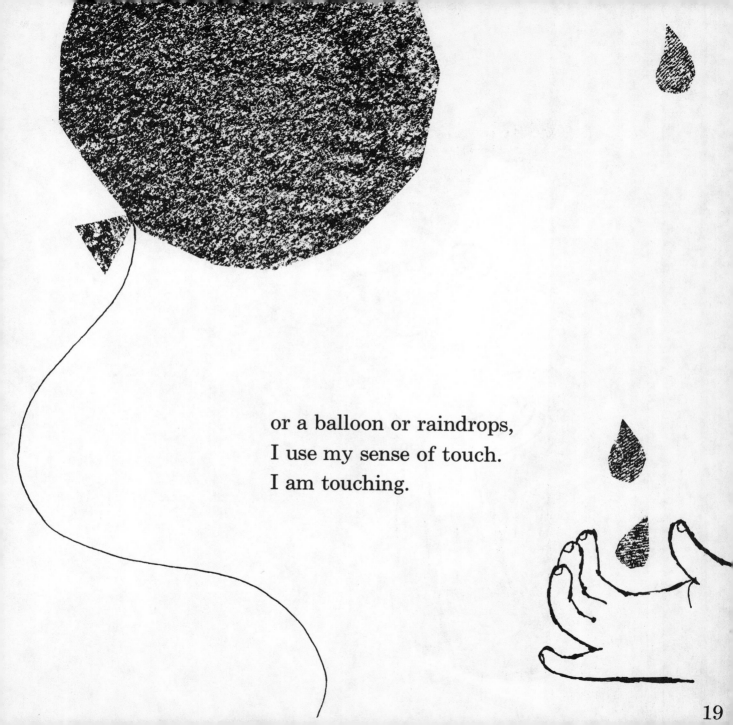

or a balloon or raindrops,
I use my sense of touch.
I am touching.

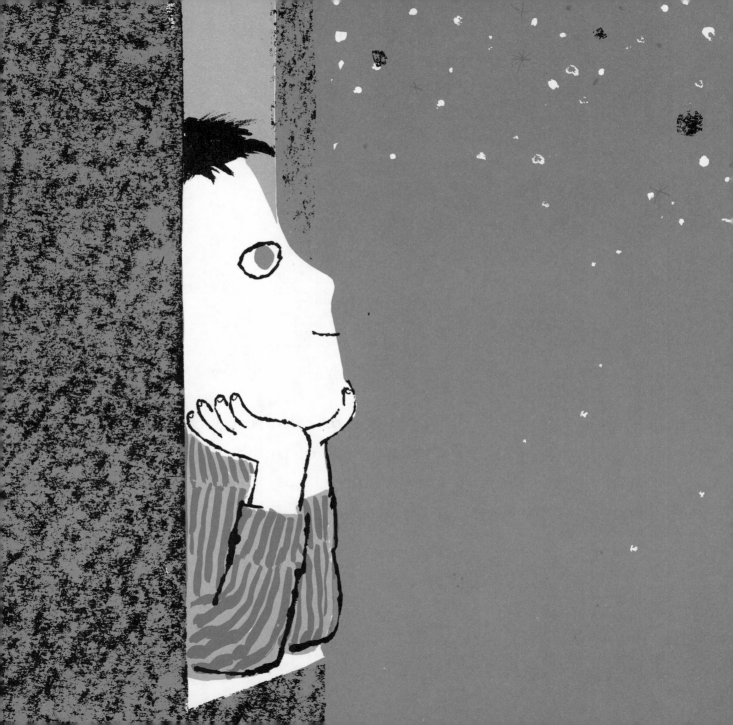

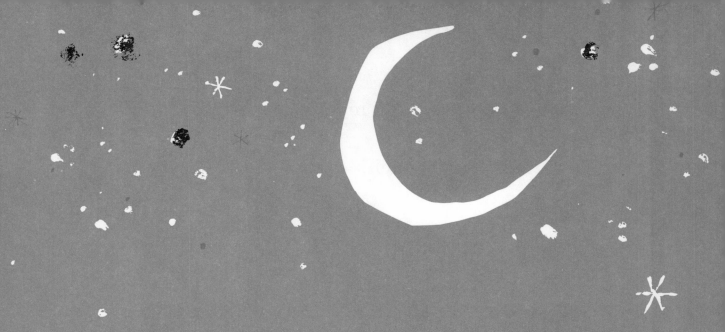

Sometimes I use all my senses at once.

Sometimes I use only one.

I often play a game with myself.

I guess how many senses I am using, at that time.

When I look at the moon and the stars,

I use one sense.

I am seeing.

When I laugh and play with my puppy,
I use four senses.
I see, hear, smell, and touch.

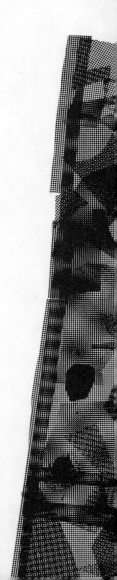

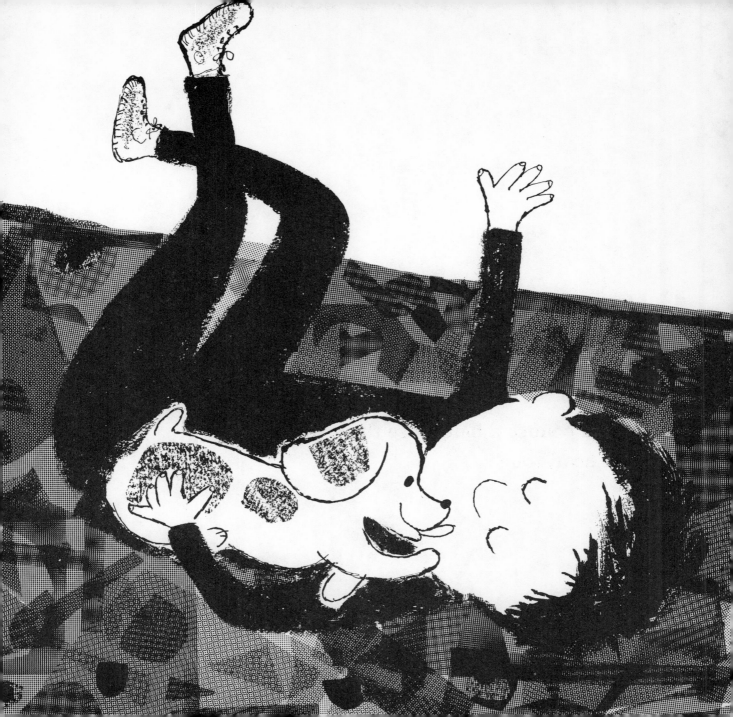

When I bounce a ball, I use three senses.
I see, hear, touch.

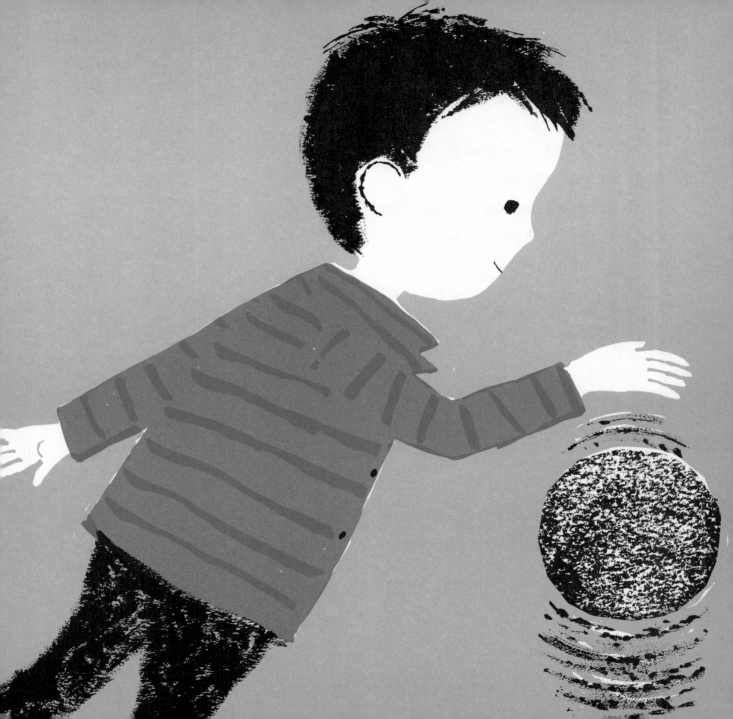

Sometimes I use more of one sense
and less of another.
But each sense is very important to me,
because it makes me aware.

To be aware is to see all there is to see . . .

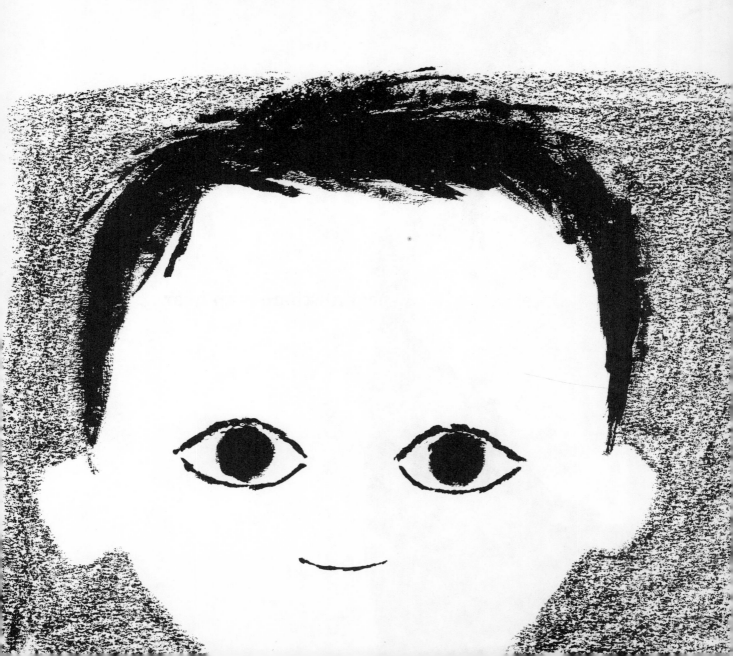

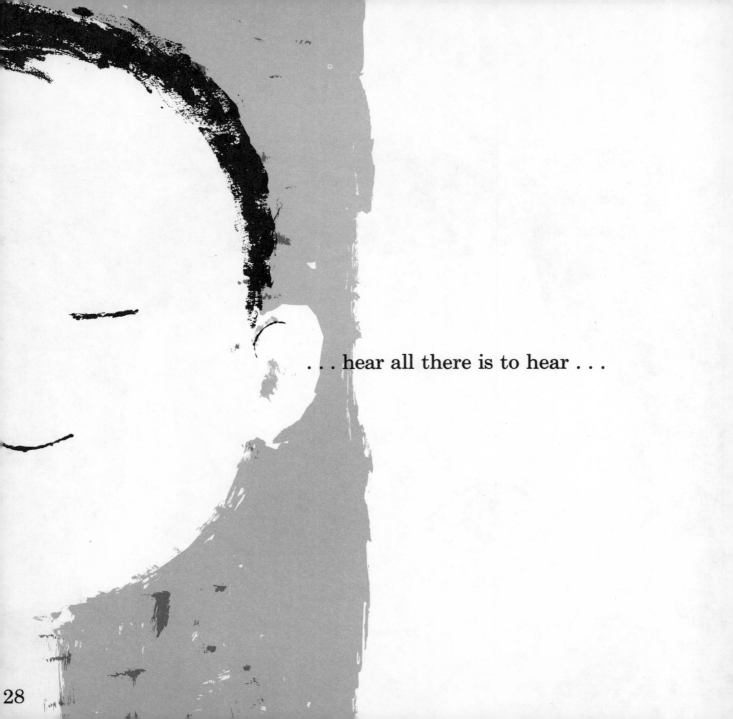

. . . hear all there is to hear . . .

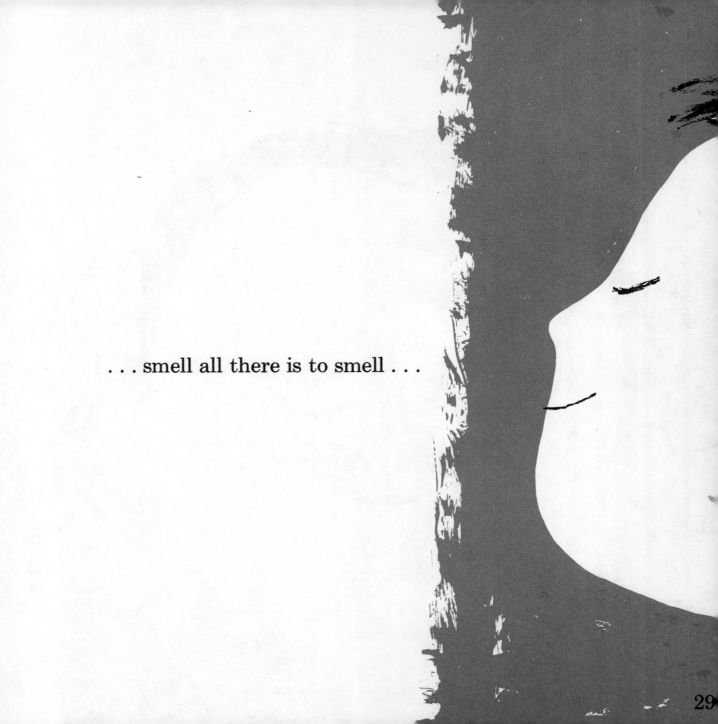

. . . smell all there is to smell . . .

29

. . . taste all there is to taste . . .

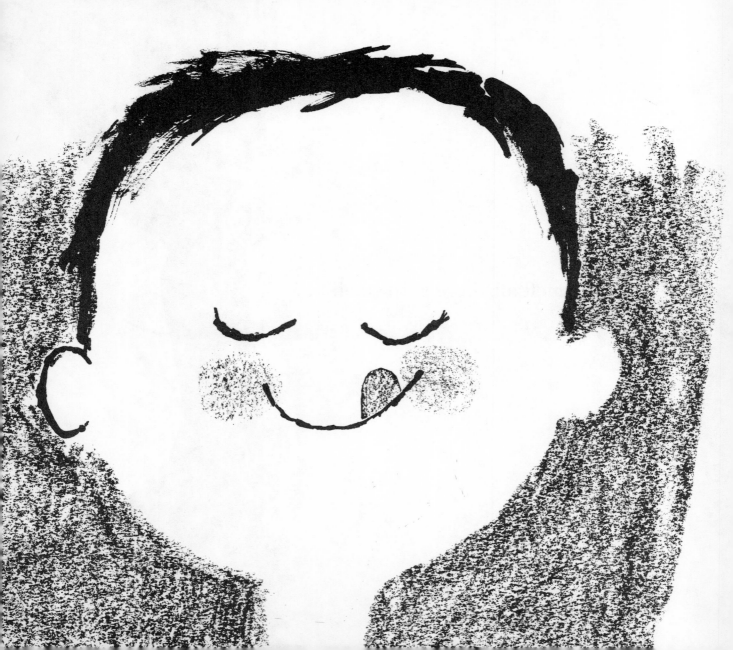

. . . touch all there is to touch.

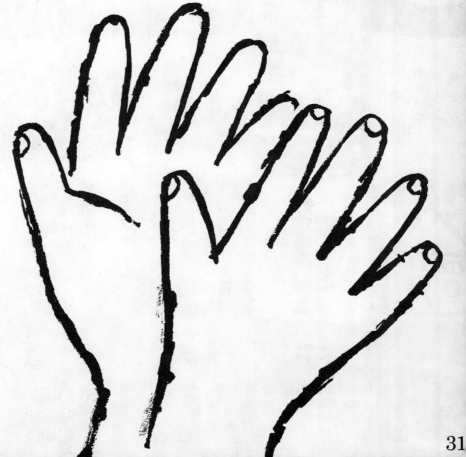

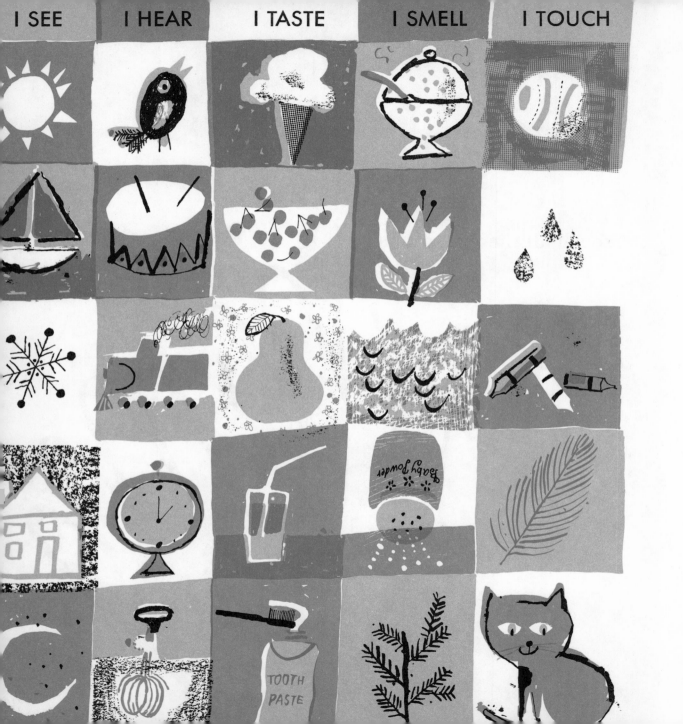

Wherever I go, whatever I do,
every minute of the day,
my senses are working.

They make me aware.

ABOUT THE AUTHOR-ILLUSTRATOR

ALIKI uses her five senses the same way she illustrates children's books and pursues commercial art—one or more at a time. She loves music, books, and watching her plants grow.

Aliki Brandenberg grew up in Philadelphia, where she attended the Museum College of Art.

Her extensive European travels include a motor and painting tour from Switzerland, where she lived and worked as an artist for four years, through Italy, Yugoslavia, and Greece.

Mr. and Mrs. Brandenberg now reside in New York City.

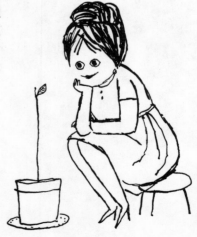